C000141447

GET FIT FAST AT HOME

Your ultimate guide to using HIIT to get leaner, stronger and fitter at home!

By Neil Cooper

GET FIT FAST AT HOME ISBN 978-1-9998728-6-1

Contents

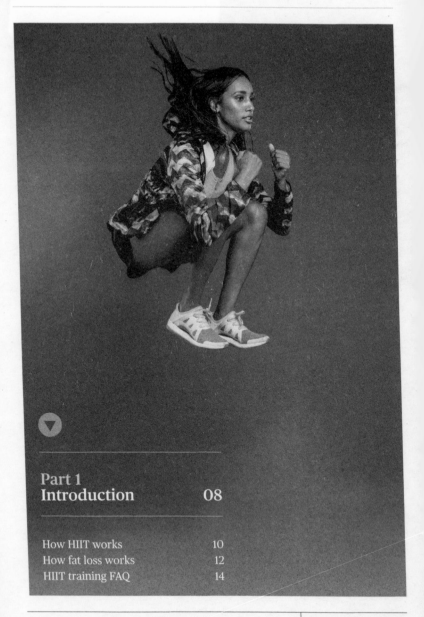

Part 1
Introduction 08

Part 2
28-Day HIIT Plan 16

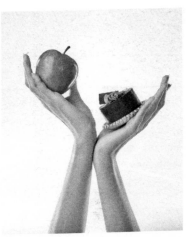

Part 4
Nutrition 72

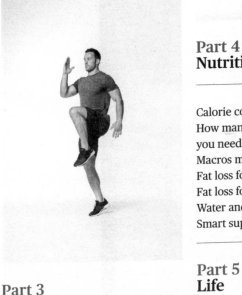

Part 3
Progression 64

Part 5
Life 90

Perfect HIIT

Welcome to your guide to losing fat for good

Welcome to *Get Fit Fast At Home: Your ultimate guide to using HIIT to get leaner, stronger and fitter at home*! We're going to start off by telling you that you've made a smart choice. Not just in buying this book, but in choosing HIIT as a way to achieve your fitness aims.

HIIT, which stands for High-Intensity Interval Training, has become increasingly popular in recent years and with good reason. It's an incredibly effective and time-efficient way of getting in shape. The fundamental reason that's the case is because working at a high intensity is demanding. And when you place a demand on your body it has no choice but to respond and rise to the challenge. This book will give you the information you need to use HIIT to get the fitness results you want.

HIIT your fitness targets

The book starts with an introduction to the concept of high-intensity interval training. We look at the theory behind the methodology, we answer some common questions, and we give you some extra tips on how to harness the power of HIIT.

Once you understand how and why HIIT works you can take on our 28-day HIIT plan. It's an accessible four-week programme that involves four quick workouts a week. Even better, you don't need any kit to do the workouts. All of the exercises in the plan are bodyweight moves, which makes it a versatile option because you can do it any time, anywhere. It's also scalable, in that you work at a rate that suits your fitness. This makes it ideal whether you're completely new to fitness or you're an experienced exerciser. The plan is set out with detailed form guides as well as bonus tips on how to maximise your progress.

Once you have completed the plan you can use the section on HIIT progressions to create your own workouts and understand the key items of home workout kit that you may want to add to your training regime.

Fast exercise, slow food

You may be familiar with the saying that "you can't out-train a bad diet". Well, that saying is absolutely true. So if you're going to use HIIT to build a better body then you'll also need to think about what you eat, both to fuel your workouts and to ensure that you recover properly too. The good news is that eating well is probably easier (and more enjoyable) than you think, and we'll give you the essential information you need to make smart choices about what you should eat and what you should avoid. We'll give you the final word on whether calories do or don't count, we'll give you a quick guide to the nutrients in key food groups, and we'll give you some easy to follow food rules that take the hassle out of healthy eating. We'll also give you a guide to the kinds of foods that you'll want to include in your diet if fat loss is your primary aim. Finally, we'll take a quick look at how drinks can affect your body shape, and we'll give you a condensed guide to sports nutrition products.

The final section in the book is devoted to the elements that often get overlooked when someone embarks upon a HIIT plan and that's the idea of rest and recovery. You see, HIIT places your body under a considerable amount of stress so it is vital that you balance that with proper recovery. The other massive but often neglected factor is sleep. Getting consistent and good quality sleep is absolutely crucial if you want to make a positive change to the way you look and feel. To finish off, we'll also give you a few expert tips on instilling good habits, so that you find it easy to make the kind of exercise, nutrition and lifestyle adjustments you need to look and feel better than ever.

Before you rush in and get moving, we'd just like you to take one more key concept on board and it is this: when it comes to exercising, quality matters. So do everything you can to make sure that your technique is flawless. It won't just help you to stay fit and injury free, it will ensure you achieve better results too.

Part 1
Introduction

Use HIIT to get fit!

One of the most important factors behind the success of any training plan is understanding the basic principles underpinning what you're doing and why you're doing it. If you have a decent grasp of those things you can start to appreciate the physical journey that you're on and you can really buy in to the process, which will also have a positive impact on your overall result.

The HIIT (high-intensity interval training) methods outlined in this book are a specific way of exercising - one that places a substantial demand on your body - so it becomes even more important that you appreciate what you're doing and how to do it. When you train at a high intensity technique is paramount, so every time you work out you must pay attention to the form guides for the exercises. You also need to be realistic about what you're going to achieve. HIIT is an incredibly effective way to train but only if you apply yourself fully to the process.

ADD IN SOME LISS
When you're doing a HIIT plan it also makes sense to add in some LISS (low-intensity steady state) work to your programme to help you recover from the high-intensity sessions and to make sure that you're not placing your body under too much stress. We'll go into more detail on this in Part 5 of the book.

How HIIT works

Here's why high-intensity training burns fat fast

WHAT IS HIIT?
HIIT stands for for High-Intensity Interval Training, and is a type of cardio activity based on doing short but intense bursts of exercise interspersed with rest periods. The key is to train at your maximum intensity for greater fat-loss results.

WHY IS HIIT SO GOOD?
HIIT is a very time-efficient way to train: working out at a high-effort levels means sessions are short, and they also burn a lot of calories, both during activity and in the hours post-training. HIIT provides closer results to weight-lifting (increased muscle mass, lower body-fat levels) than traditional types of cardio, like jogging.

DON'T HIIT SESSIONS REQUIRE LOTS OF RUNNING?
HIIT sessions don't have to be based on sprinting or running: you can use weights to perform a HIIT session: for example, doing multiple moves in a circuit to get your heart rate high and work all your main muscle groups to burn calories and add lean size.

WHAT ELSE DO I NEED TO KNOW?
You should limit how much HIIT you do per week. Too much can cause fatigue and your progress to stall, so always use it wisely.

Common HIIT session formats

There are lots of HIIT protocols you could deploy to elicit the fat-burning and muscle-building response you want - in many ways you are only limited by the equipment at hand and your imagination. To help you find your feet, here are some of the most common and popular forms of HIIT protocols, some of which feature later in this book.

Circuits
Circuits are a combination of different moves done back-to-back with little or no rest between exercises, and a longer rest between each circuit, or "round". There can be any number of moves, but usually at least four. Circuits also typically use the same equipment: a barbell circuit is called a barbell "complex".

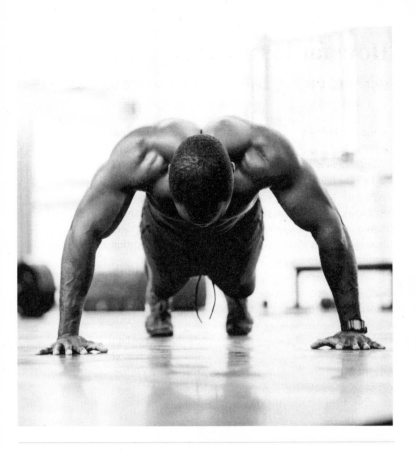

NEAT

NEAT stands for "non-exercise activity thermogenesis", and accounts for all the calories you burn each day through "living life", so walking, moving around the office, and fidgeting. While exercise has the biggest impact on fat loss, the more you move every day the more total calories you burn.

SLEEP

Sleep, along with stress, are the two factors most people neglect to consider when wanting to lose weight, but getting enough high-quality sleep each night will go a huge way towards building a better body. Aim for 7-9 hours a night, and keep your bedroom as dark and cool as possible.

STRESS

Acute - or long-term - stress is very damaging to your health, negatively impacting hormomes, appetite, motivation and many areas of your life. Minimise stress by finding ways to relax daily, because the less stressed you are, the more energy you'll have and the faster you'll lose fat.

HIIT training FAQ

Do I have to be fit to start?
No - the beauty of HIIT is that you only ever exercise at your own upper capability: that means your effort level is always relative to your fitness level. For example, someone very new to HIIT may only be able to do five burpees in a minute, whereas someone very experienced may do 20. However, because both are working at their top capacity they'll both reap the benefits.

What happens if I can't complete a workout?
It is possible to complete workouts, however, you may just need to rest for slightly longer between exercises and/or rounds. This may require some trial and error, but begin by sticking to the rest periods detailed in the workout chapter. If it's not long enough for you to adequately recover, then increase each rest period by five seconds. Keep doing this until you find the right amount of recovery time (but remember to decrease it as you become fitter).

When will I start seeing results?
Everyone is different so will start noticing positive adaptations to their physiques and fitness levels at different rates. However, if you follow the plan to the letter and push yourself in each and every session, then you'll amaze yourself at how quickly you start to look, feel and perform better.

Is HIIT the only kind of training I need?
HIIT is one of the most efficient and effective training protocols for burning fat and building muscle, so should form the backbone of any better-body training programme. But that's not to say other forms of exercise, such as low-intensity, steady-state (LISS) cardio like jogging or cycling aren't beneficial. While they might not ramp up your body's calorie-burning capabilities as much as HIIT or weight-lifting, they can provide a huge mental boost, which will only increase your confidence and motivation.

Can I eat what I want?
What you eat can be as important as how you exercise when wanting to get lean, and the old saying that "you can't out-train a bad diet" still rings true. To get leaner faster base your meals on lean meat and fish, plenty of fresh fruit and veg, and carbs in their natural form, such as rice and potatoes. You should also cut back on sugar (especially in soft drinks, chocolate and biscuits), limit alcohol intake, and avoid highly-processed snacks.

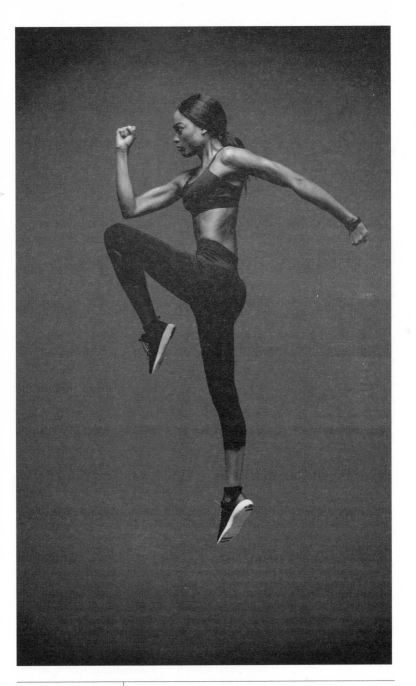

Part 2
Your 28-day HIIT plan

Four weeks to a fitter, healthier and happier you!

You're nearly ready to start your 28-day HIIT programme. All you need to do is have a quick read of the following pages and then put the plan into action.

The programme we've created is progressive, meaning it gets harder as you get fitter. We've considered all of the potential workout variables (such as number of exercises, quantity of rounds and length of rest) to create a fast and effective routine. And that's why the closer you follow the plan, the better your results will be.

The other thing we're asking you to do is to commit to each session because the more effort you put in to each workout, the better your outcome will be. The sessions themselves are relatively short - you'll be done in about 20-30 minutes. That doesn't mean that they are easy, and this kind of training can get deceptively tough quickly. But if you dig deep and power on through to the finish, we promise that your body will soon be flooding with feel-good endorphins.

PERFECT FORM
You may be familiar with the idea of exercise "form". It refers to the technique you use to perform an exercise. Maintaining good form matters because if you do an exercise correctly then you'll recruit the target muscles effectively and you'll get the desired result. If your form is sloppy then you may end up using momentum, rather than your muscles, to power the exercise. That might make you feel good in the moment but it won't make you look good in the long run.

How the plan works

Here's what you need to know about your plan

STICK TO THE PLAN

We've considered all the specifics of the plan, so your only job is simply to execute the workouts as they appear in the workout tables. It's really important that you do the workouts in order and the exercises in the order that they appear in order to elicit the desired physiological response. We also advise against second guessing your progress and adding in extra moves to speed things up because longer workouts don't automatically mean better results.

THINK IN BLOCKS

The 28-day plan is split up into four week-long blocks. Each block is composed of workouts that follow the same structure. The reason the block formats change is to ensure that you challenge yourself, rather than seeing your progress stall.

WORKOUT TABLES

Follow the tables for each session as closely as possible. You'll notice that different workouts have different formats but the key things to look out for are outlined opposite.

REST DAYS

There are four workouts a week and you should generally aim to have a rest day between workouts. Of course, you can't do four workouts and have four rest days in a week so you will have to do two of the workouts on consecutive days. So, for example, you could do Monday, Wednesday, Friday and Saturday. Or, if you want to keep the weekend free, you can do Monday, Tuesday, Thursday and Friday. The best time of day to do the workouts is the time you can stick to. Just be aware that if you do the workouts in the evening that may impact your sleep because exercising with intensity will excite your central nervous system, which may make it difficult for you to fall asleep quickly.

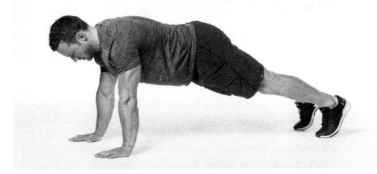

Workout tables decoded

Exercise name	R1	R2	R3	R4	Rest
1. Split squat (left)	20s	20s	20s	20s	10s
2. Incline press-up	20s	20s	20s	20s	10s
3. Split squat (right)	20s	20s	20s	20s	10s
4. Run on the spot	20s	20s	20s	20s	10s
5. Crunch	20s	20s	20s	20s	60s

Exercise name
Do the exercises in order as they appear in the workouts. Pay close attention to the 'How to do it' section that accompanies each workout, and also the form guides that give you the correct technique for each exercise.

Rounds
Next to the exercise name you'll see column with 'R1', 'R2' and so on at the top. 'R' stands for 'round' and you should perform the designated time or reps for each exercise in order to complete one round. Do as many rounds as are indicated in the workout table.

Rest
The final column may include details about how long you should rest after each exercise and between rounds. It's really important that you stick to this time if you want to get the desired training effect. Resting for too long, for example, reduces the intensity (and the effectiveness) of your session.

Performance-boosting tips

Use these tips to accelerate your progress

You can have the best workout in the world on paper, but there's one vital ingredient that brings it to life and makes it work - and that's you. There are three main things you can do to maximise the results you see from your plan. The first is to stick to it as closely as possible, which should be pretty easy to do. The next is to apply as much effort as you can to each session. You can think of this as a skill in itself and it is something that you'll have to work on over time. But be very clear - you will get out what you put in, so take that as a positive. The more you put in, the more you'll get out. The final thing is to use some extra techniques and tactics, such as those outlined below.

Smart workout tactics

MASTER TECHNIQUE
Before you begin your programme it makes sense to familiarise yourself with the correct exercise technique so that you can attack each session with confidence. It may be useful to have a couple of practise sessions where you make sure that you're happy with all of the exercises in the plan.

USE VISUALISATION
There is strong scientific evidence to suggest that using basic visualisation techniques can improve your outcome. For example, before your workout, spend a minute getting in the zone by picturing yourself performing each move with perfect form.

MIND AND MUSCLE
This is a technique you can borrow from bodybuilders, who use the 'mind to muscle connection' concept to boost their results. You may not want to look like a bodybuilder but you're probably keen to fast-track your progress. Just think about the target muscle as you perform each rep.

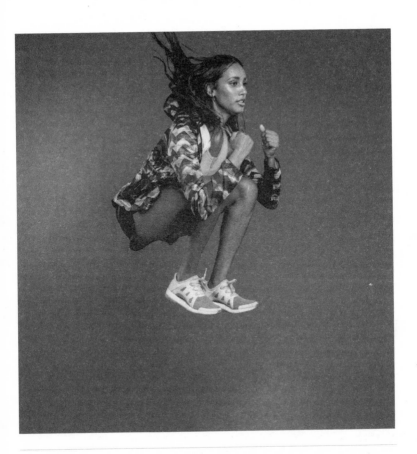

CONTROL YOUR INNER VOICE
It's highly likely that your mind will want to give up before your body is ready to give in. We've all experienced that 'inner voice' when exercising that tells us to stop. Your job is to silence that voice. It's not necessarily easy to do but it will make a huge difference to your results.

DO ONE MORE REP
When you think that you've done all you can, try to do one more rep. Whether you complete that extra rep doesn't really mater. The important element is that you try to do it, because that extra effort will help you to squeeze every last ounce of capacity out of your muscles.

BE YOUR OWN COACH
Imagine that you were doing your workout and you had an elite coach watching over you and assisting with your session. Would you give up easily? Or would their presence help you to push yourself even harder? It's a simple but effective technique that helps to ensure that your effort levels remain high.

Record your performance

Keep track to stay on track for success

If you don't record what you do in your workouts then how will you ever really know if you're making progress? After all, can you remember how many reps you did of a particular exercise in a workout a few weeks ago? We thought not. And that's why keeping a simple record of what you've done is so important. In fact, it's one of the most effective ways to stay motivated and keep moving forwards. Almost all fitness progress requires a huge physical and mental effort so you'd be daft to pass on the opportunity to take advantage of something that's so helpful and so easy to do.

Our advice is to get a notebook or a dedicated workout journal, and fill it out between sets. If you've never done this before, ensure that you fill out the basic workout details as an absolute minimum and, if you can, try to include other items of information as outlined below.

BASIC INFO
In this instance, we'd like you to record the reps that you do of each of the moves in each workout. If you do other programmes in future, you should continue to note this basic workout information. Other programmes might require you to record extra information, such as the tempo (speed) of each rep but for now we can keep it relatively simple.

NUTRITION INFO
You don't need to keep a comprehensive food diary but it can be useful to record what you eat before, during and after your sessions so that you can assess how your nutrition intake is affecting your performance. Write down what and how much you eat before your workout, as well as any pre-workout vitamins or supplements. You should also record how much water you drink during a session, any sports nutrition drinks or products you consume during your session, and what you eat for your post-workout meal.

EXTRA ANALYSIS
If you're really enjoying the process of recording your workout performance and nutrition, you can add even more detail, which will help you to build a really comprehensive picture of the factors that are influencing your rate of progress. If, however, you're finding it difficult to record the basics, there's no point in over-burdening yourself. But if you are up for it, write down the time of the workout and how much sleep you got the night before, and rate your quality of sleep out of ten. After each session, note what went well, what could be improved and anything that you'll try to do differently next time to boost your performance.

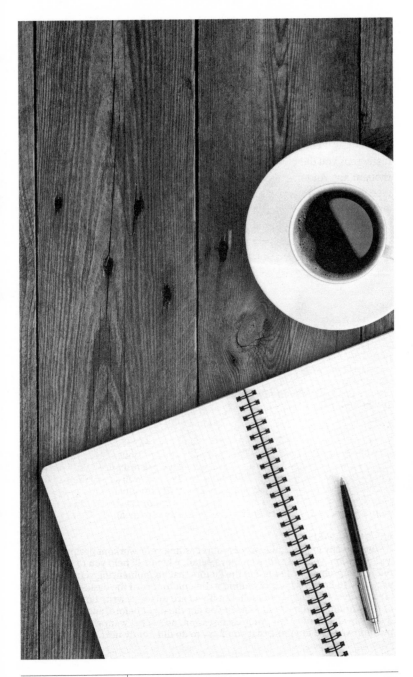

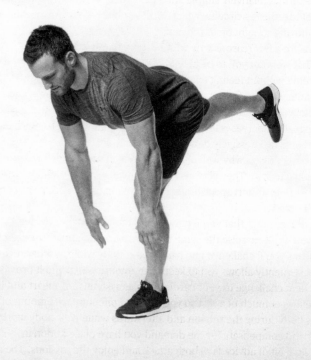

Week 1

You're now ready to start your four-week HIIT programme. This week we've kept the format relatively simple and you'll perform four workouts that have been put together as circuits, which means you do one set of an exercise before moving straight on to the next exercise with minimal rest.

There are a few reasons why we've used this approach in week 1. The first is that we want you to be able to make a quick and easy start to your programme without feeling overwhelmed by a complex session structure. This simple workout format allows you to devote all of your effort and energy to executing the exercises to the best of your ability. And as your fitness capacity increases during the course of the four weeks, we'll make the workouts progressively demanding.

The other reason why we've gone for circuits is because they are incredibly effective. They allow you to complete a large volume of good quality work in a short space of time, meaning that you get a great bang for your HIIT buck.

One of the things that you'll notice in all of the workouts during this week is that you don't exercise the same muscle groups in concurrent exercises. That means you'll challenge one part of your body while another recovers. This subsequently allows you to keep your intensity high and it provides an excellent challenge to your cardiovascular system. Your heart and lungs don't really get much of a rest so you'll burn a phenomenal amount of calories both during the session and afterwards while your body works to recover and compensate for the demand you have placed upon it.

Our final bit of advice is to both attack and enjoy the sessions. The more you put into them, the more you'll get out of it. So give each exercise in each round your 100% effort and you'll be astonished by how amazing you'll feel.

Week 1 *Workout 1*

⏱ Time **20 mins**   ⬌ Format **Circuit**

Exercise name	R1	R2	R3	R4	Rest
1. Split squat (left)	20s	20s	20s	20s	10s
2. Incline press-up	20s	20s	20s	20s	10s
3. Split squat (right)	20s	20s	20s	20s	10s
4. Standing sprint	20s	20s	20s	20s	10s
5. Crunch	20s	20s	20s	20s	60s

Workout format and form guides

HOW TO DO IT
Do as many reps as you can in 20 seconds of exercise 1 then rest for 10 seconds before doing as many reps as you can of exercise 2 and so on until you have done each of the five exercises. That's one round. At the end of each round rest for 60 seconds and complete four rounds in total.

1. Split squat (left)
Stand tall with your left foot forward and your chest up and abs engaged. Bend both knees to lunge down until your right knee almost touches the floor. Push through your left foot to return to the start and repeat.

2. Incline press-up
Get into the press-up position with your hands under your shoulders on a box or raised platform. Your body should form a straight line from head to heels. Engage your abs and bend your elbows to lower your chest towards the floor. Go as low as you can, then press back up to straighten your arms and return to the start position.

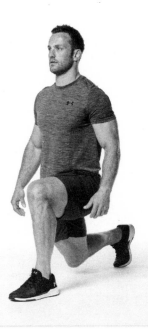

3. Split squat (right)
Stand tall with your right foot forward and your chest up and abs engaged. Bend both knees to lunge down until your left knee almost touches the floor. Push through your right foot to return to the start and repeat.

4. Standing sprint
Stand tall with your chest up and abs engaged. Sprint on the spot, raising your knees as high as possible and swinging your arms back and forth.

5. Crunch
Lie flat on your back with your knees bent and feet flat on the floor, and bend your arms so your fingers touch the side of your head. Engage your abs, then raise your torso off the floor without tensing your neck. Keep that tension on your abs as you slowly lower your torso back to the floor.

Week 1 *Workout 2*

⏱ Time **20 mins**   ⬡ Format **Circuit**

Exercise name	R1	R2	R3	R4	Rest
1. Lunge	20s	20s	20s	20s	10s
2. Press-up	20s	20s	20s	20s	10s
3. Squat	20s	20s	20s	20s	10s
4. High knees	20s	20s	20s	20s	10s
5. Reverse crunch	20s	20s	20s	20s	60s

Workout format and form guides

HOW TO DO IT
Do as many reps as you can in 20 seconds of exercise 1 then rest for 10 seconds before doing as many reps as you can of exercise 2 and so on until you have done each of the five exercises. That's one round. At the end of each round rest for 60 seconds and complete four rounds in total.

1. Lunge
Stand with your chest up, abs engaged and arms by your sides. Take a big step forwards with your left foot, then bend both knees to lunge down until your right knee almost touches the floor. Push through your left foot to return to the start, then step forwards with your right foot and repeat the move, alternating leading legs with each rep.

2. Press-up
Get into the press-up position with your legs and arms straight, and your hands under your shoulders. Your body should form a straight line from head to heels. Bend your elbows to lower your chest towards the floor. Go as low as you can, then press back up to straighten your arms and return to the start position.

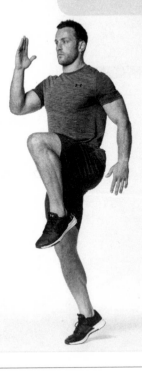

3. Squat
Stand tall with your chest up, abs engaged and arms straight by your sides. Bend your knees to squat down as low as you can, either keeping your arms by your sides or raising them up to shoulder height. Push through your heels to straighten your legs and return to the start position.

4. High knees
Stand tall with your chest up and abs engaged. Start sprinting on the spot, swinging your arms and bringing your knees up as high as possible. You can also put your arms out straight in front of you and try to make your knees hit your palms with each step.

5. Reverse crunch
Lie flat on your back with knees bent and feet on the floor. Place your arms by your sides. Engage your lower abs then raise your heels off the floor. Keeping your core tight, use your lower abs to raise your knees up and in towards your chest. Hold the top position for a second then lower your feet back to the floor.

Week 1 *Workout 3*

⏱ Time **20 mins**　　　　　🔘 Format **Circuit**

Exercise name	R1	R2	R3	R4	Rest
1. Lunge reach	20s	20s	20s	20s	10s
2. Wide press-up	20s	20s	20s	20s	10s
3. Pause squat	20s	20s	20s	20s	10s
4. Mountain climber	20s	20s	20s	20s	10s
5. Leg raise	20s	20s	20s	20s	60s

Workout format and form guides

HOW TO DO IT
Do as many reps as you can of exercise 1 then rest in 20 seconds for 10 seconds before doing as many reps as you can of exercise 2 and so on until you have done each of the five exercises. That's one round. At the end of each round rest for 60 seconds and complete four rounds in total.

1. Lunge reach
Stand with your chest up, abs engaged and arms straight above your head. Take a big step forwards with your left foot and bend both knees to lunge down while leaning over to your left. Push through your front foot to return to the start, then step forwards with your right foot and repeat the move, leaning to your right. Alternate sides each rep.

2. Wide press-up
Get into the press-up position but with your hands double shoulder-width apart. Your body should form a straight line from head to heels. Engage your abs and bend your elbows to lower your chest towards the floor. Go as low as you can, then press back up to straighten your arms and return to the start position.

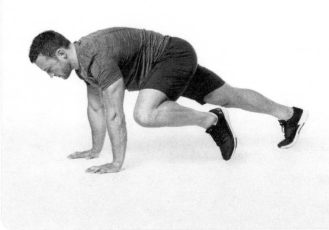

3. Pause squat
Bend your knees to squat down as low as you can, bringing your arms out in front of you to shoulder height. Keep your chest up and abs engaged and maintain this position. If you start to struggle, stand back up, take two deep breaths, then squat back down and hold.

4. Mountain climber
Get on all fours with your arms and legs straight and your wrists directly under your shoulders. Without letting your hips sag, draw one knee up and bring it towards the elbow on the same side. Straighten that leg, then repeat, bringing your other knee towards your elbow. Keep your abs engaged and keep the reps fast but controlled.

5. Leg raise
Lie flat on your back with your legs straight. Engage your abs, then raise your feet off the floor. Keeping your legs straight, raise your feet as high as you can, then slowly lower them. You can make the move harder and work your lower abs more by not allowing your heels to touch the floor between reps.

Week 1 *Workout 4*

Exercise name	R1	R2	R3	R4	Rest
1. Single leg RDL (left)	20s	20s	20s	20s	10s
2. Decline press-up	20s	20s	20s	20s	10s
3. Single leg RDL (right)	20s	20s	20s	20s	10s
4. Jumping jacks	20s	20s	20s	20s	10s
5. Bicycle	20s	20s	20s	20s	60s

Workout format and form guides

HOW TO DO IT
Do as many reps as you can in 20 seconds of exercise 1 then rest for 10 seconds before doing as many reps as you can of exercise 2 and so on until you have done each of the five exercises. That's one round. At the end of each round rest for 60 seconds and complete four rounds in total.

1. Single leg RDL (left)
Stand tall on your left leg with your chest up, abs engaged and arms straight out in front of you. With a slight bend in your left knee, bend forwards from the hips then reach your fingertips down as far as possible, raising your right leg behind you for balance. Return to the start position and repeat.

2. Decline press-up
Get into the press-up position but with your feet on a box or raised platform. Your body should form a straight line from head to heels. Engage your abs and bend your elbows to lower your chest towards the floor. Go as low as you can, then press back up to straighten your arms and return to the start position.

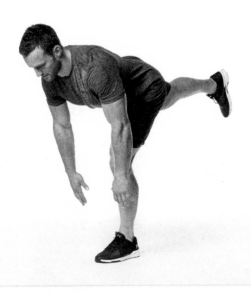

3. Single leg RDL (left)
Stand tall on your right leg with your chest up, abs engaged and arms straight out in front of you. With a slight bend in your right knee, bend forwards from the hips then reach your fingertips down as far as possible, raising your right leg behind you for balance. Return to the start position and repeat.

4. Jumping jacks
Stand tall with your chest up, abs engaged and hands by your sides. Jump up and bring both feet out wide to the sides while raising your arms to the sides so your hands finish above your head. Jump back from the wide stance to the start position, lowering your arms as you go.

5. Bicycle
Lie on your back with your hands by your head and legs straight. Raise your torso and feet and engage your abs. Crunch up and rotate your torso to one side, bringing in your opposite knee to touch your elbow. Reverse the move back to the start (without your back or feet touching the floor), then repeat, alternating sides each rep.

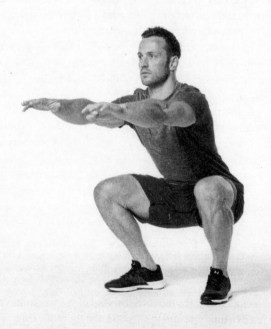

Week 2

Congratulations on completing week one. In many ways you've done the hardest week. It's so easy to come up with an excuse not to start but you've taken the initiative and you've powered through your first week. Let's now use that positive momentum to make this week even better.

In the first week we kept things pretty simple with some full-body circuits. In this week we get a bit more creative to ensure that your mind is engaged and we challenge your muscles and cardiovascular system in a fresh and effective way.

All of the workouts in this week use what's known as a '6, 12, 25' structure in a mini-circuit format. That means you do six reps of exercise 1a, take a very short rest, perform 12 moves of exercise 1b, take a very short rest and perform 25 reps of exercise 1c. All three exercises will focus on the same body part, which poses a huge challenge to your muscles because the high number of total reps will mean that they start to fatigue and you'll really have to fight through to the finish.

An important element in the session design for this week is that the hardest of the three moves goes first and the easiest goes third. That way you'll be able to complete the workouts. If we asked you to do 25 reps of the hardest exercise, it's unlikely that you'd be able to get anywhere near the end of the workout.

We've also included two abs moves at the end of the workout. The first of these moves is a dynamic one and the second one is a static exercise. That's a great combination because it will challenge your abs and core in two very different but very effective ways.

As ever, we'd like you to give 100% effort to each session. And think about this - at the end of the week you'll be half way through the plan and that's when you can start to think about being in the home straight.

Week 2 *Workout 1*

⏱ Time **20 mins**　　　　　🎛 Format **6, 12, 25**

Exercise name	R1	R2	R3	Rest
1a. Lunge jump	6	6	6	10s
1b. Reverse lunge	12	12	12	10s
1c. Lunge	25	25	25	90s
2. Crunch reach	12	12	12	30s
3. Tall plank	30s	30s	30s	60s

Workout format and form guides

HOW TO DO IT
**Do 6 reps of exercise
1a, then rest for 10 secs.
Do 12 reps of exercise
1b then rest for 10 secs.
Do 25 reps of exercise
1c then rest for 90 secs.
Do 12 reps of exercise
2 then rest for 30 secs
before doing 30 secs of
exercise 3 to complete
one round. Do 3
rounds in total, resting
for 60 secs between
rounds.**

1a. Lunge jump
Stand with your chest up, abs engaged and feet hip-width apart. Take a big step forwards with your left foot, then bend both knees to lunge down. Push through your front foot to jump into the air, switching legs mid-air, so you land with your right foot forward. Go straight into another lunge and repeat, switching your leading leg in the air.

1b. Reverse lunge
Stand tall with your chest up, abs engaged and arms by your sides. Take a big step backwards with your left foot, then bend both knees to lunge down. Push through your back foot to return to the start, then step backwards with your right foot and repeat the move. Alternate sides with each rep.

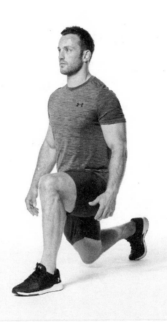

BONUS TIP: Ahead of each round, take three very deep breaths and think about your goals to really focus your mind.

1c. Lunge
Stand tall with your chest up, abs engaged and arms by your sides. Take a big step forwards with your left foot, then bend both knees to lunge down until your right knee almost touches the floor. Push through your left foot to return to the start, then step forwards with your right foot and repeat the move, alternating leading legs each rep.

2. Crunch reach
Lie flat on your back with knees bent and arms straight and pointing up. Engage your abs to raise your torso up as high as you can, while reaching upwards towards the ceiling. Hold this top position for a second, then lower your torso back to the start. Make it harder by not allowing your upper back to touch the floor between reps.

3. Tall plank
Get into the press-up position with your palms on the floor, your wrists underneath your shoulders and your body in a straight line from head to heels. Keep your abs and glutes fully engaged to hold this position without letting your hips sag, and keep your breathing controlled.

Week 2 *Workout 2*

⏱ Time **20 mins**　　　　　　◑ Format **6, 12, 25**

Exercise name	R1	R2	R3	Rest
1a. Press-up	6	6	6	10s
1b. Incline press-up	12	12	12	10s
1c. Eccentric press-up	25	25	25	90s
2. V-up	12	12	12	30s
3. Plank	30s	30s	30s	60s

Workout format and form guides

HOW TO DO IT
Do 6 reps of exercise
1a, then rest for 10 secs.
Do 12 reps of exercise
1b then rest for 10 secs.
Do 25 reps of exercise
1c then rest for 90 secs.
Do 12 reps of exercise
2 then rest for 30 secs
before doing 30 secs of
exercise 3 to complete
one round. Do 3
rounds in total, resting
for 60 secs between
rounds.

1a. Press-up
Get into the press-up
position with your legs
and arms straight, and
your hands under your
shoulders. Your body
should form a straight
line from head to heels.
Engage your abs and
bend your elbows to
lower your chest towards
the floor. Go as low as
you can, then press up to
straighten your arms and
return to the start.

1b. Incline press-up
Start in the press-up position but with your hands
under your shoulders on
a box or raised platform.
Your body should form
a straight line from head
to heels. Engage your abs
and bend your elbows to
lower your chest towards
the floor. Go as low as
you can, then press back
up to straighten your
arms and return to the
start position.

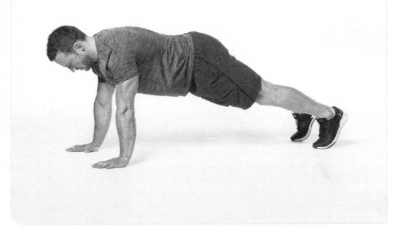

BONUS TIP: If you struggle to engage your abs draw your belly button towards your spine - as if you were about to take a punch.

1c. Eccentric press-up

Start in the press-up position with your body straight. Engage your abs and bend your elbows to lower your chest towards the floor as slowly as possible. Once at the bottom, let your chest touch the floor, then go on to your knees to help yourself return to the start position. Repeat these slow, down-only reps.

2. V-up

Lie flat on your back with your legs straight and your arms straight pointing behind you. Engage your abs and with your arms and legs straight, raise your arms and feet off the floor, and bring your arms forwards so your hands touch your legs. Reach as far up your leg as possible. Reverse the move to return to the start.

3. Plank

Get into the plank position, supporting yourself on your forearms with your elbows underneath your shoulders. Engage your abs, then raise your hips off the floor so that your body forms a straight line from head to heels. Hold this position without letting your hips sag, and keep your breathing controlled.

Week 2 *Workout 3*

⏱ Time **20 mins**   ⊕⊕ Format **6, 12, 25**

Exercise name	R1	R2	R3	Rest
1a. Squat jump	6	6	6	10s
1b. 1 and 1/4 squat	12	12	12	10s
1c. Squat	25	25	25	90s
2. Russian twist	12	12	12	30s
3. Side plank (each side)	15s	15s	15s	60s

Workout format and form guides

HOW TO DO IT
Do 6 reps of exercise
1a, then rest for 10 secs.
Do 12 reps of exercise
1b then rest for 10 secs.
Do 25 reps of exercise
1c then rest for 90 secs.
Do 12 reps of exercise
2 then rest for 30 secs
before doing 15 secs of
exercise 3 each side to
complete one round.
Do 3 rounds in total,
resting for 60 secs
between rounds.

1a. Squat jump
Stand tall with your chest
up, abs engaged and
arms straight by your
sides. Bend your knees
to squat down as low as
you can, and swing your
arms backwards. Push
through your heels to
straighten your legs and
jump powerfully off the
floor. Land on both feet
and go straight into the
next rep.

1b. 1 and 1/4 squat
Stand with your chest up,
abs engaged and arms
straight by your sides.
Bend your knees to squat
down as low as you can,
either keeping your arms
by your sides or raising
them to shoulder height.
From the bottom position
of the squat, come back
up one-quarter of the
way to standing back up,
then squat down before
then standing up fully.

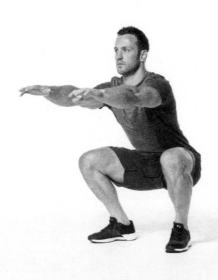

BONUS TIP: Keep your intensity up by doing each rep fast, yet controlled, to work your heart, lungs and muscles harder.

1c. Squat
Stand tall with your chest up, abs engaged and arms straight by your sides. Bend your knees to squat down as low as you can, either keeping your arms by your sides or raising them up to shoulder height. Push through your heels to straighten your legs and return to the start position.

2. Russian twist
Sit up with your chest up, abs engaged and a slight bend in your knees. Use your abs to rotate your torso to one side, then return to the middle and rotate to the other side. Make the move harder by raising your heels off the floor and keeping them raised.

3. Side plank
Lie on your left-hand side, supported by your left forearm, with your right arm against your right side, and your left foot on the floor. Engage your core and glutes then raise your hips up so your body is straight from head to heels. Hold this position without letting your hips sag for the stated time, then swap sides and repeat.

Week 2 *Workout 4*

⏱ Time **20 mins**   ⬦ Format **6, 12, 25**

Exercise name	R1	R2	R3	Rest
1a. Glute bridge	6	6	6	10s
1b. Single leg RDL reach	12	12	12	10s
1c. RDL	25	25	25	90s
2. Thread the needle	12	12	12	30s
3. Side plank star (each side)	15s	15s	15s	60s

Workout format and form guides

HOW TO DO IT
Do 6 reps of exercise 1a, then rest for 10 secs. Do 12 reps of exercise 1b then rest for 10 secs. Do 25 reps of exercise 1c then rest for 90 secs. Do 12 reps of exercise 2 then rest for 30 secs before doing 15 secs of exercise 3 each side to complete one round. Do 3 rounds in total, resting for 60 secs between rounds.

1a. Glute bridge
Lie flat on your back with your hands on your stomach and your knees bent. Engage your abs and your glutes, then raise your hips off the floor. Squeeze your glutes hard at the top, then lower your hips to return to the start position.

1b. Single-leg RDL reach
Stand on your left leg with your chest up, abs engaged and arms straight out in front of you. With a slight bend in your left knee, bend forwards from the hips then reach your fingertips forwards as far as possible, raising your right leg behind you for balance. Return to the start and repeat for the stated time.

BONUS TIP: Stay hydrated by drinking water at the end of each round. You don't need much: just a few big sips.

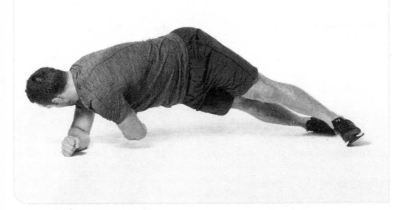

1c. RDL

Stand tall with your chest up, abs engaged and arms straight by your sides. With a slight bend in your knees, bend forwards from the hips then reach your fingertips down the front of your legs as far as possible, until you feel a good stretch in your hamstrings. Return to the start position and repeat.

2. Thread the needle

Get into position, supporting yourself on your forearms with your elbows underneath your shoulders. Lift one hand off the floor. Rotate your torso and raise that arm. Rotate back down and move that arm underneath your body, then rotate back again. Do the stated number of reps, then repeat on your other side.

3. Side plank star

Lie on your left-hand side, supported by your left forearm. Engage your core and glutes then raise your hips up so your body is straight from head to heels. Then raise your right leg and right arm up into the air as high as you can. Hold this position without letting your hips sag for the stated number of reps, swap sides and repeat.

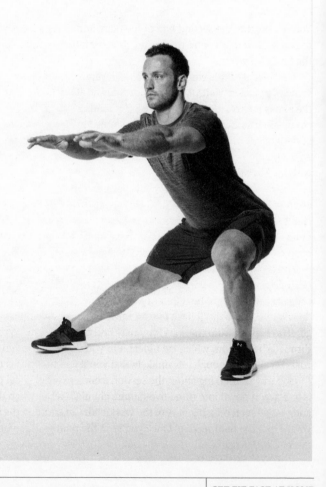

Week 3

You're now into the second half of the plan, and that's a massive milestone to reach. Now that you're this far in, you owe it to yourself to power through the final two weeks.

The format of this week's sessions is deceptively simple. It uses something called AMRAP, which stands for As Many Rounds As Possible, and the aim is for you to complete as many rounds as you can of the outlined circuits in just 15 minutes. But don't be fooled by the simplicity. The absence of designated rest periods means that you're supposed to keep going for the entire 15 minutes and that is a substantial length of time to be working for without a break.

The reason this is in week three is because it wouldn't really be appropriate to chuck it in earlier because it provides such a big fitness challenge. One of the secrets to a good exercise programme is keeping you motivated and feeling good about your sessions. If we threw you in at the deep end then you'd just get demoralised and you might give up.

The other thing that's great about this kind of session is that it will be done according to your ability. Your job is to work at your maximum capacity and that will be different for everyone. The crucial thing is that you do what you can. You'll have to experiment a bit with how fast you should go. If you sprint from the start, you may find that you need to rest halfway through the session, which isn't ideal. But you don't want to go too slow and coast through (although it is unlikely that you'll feel that this is too easy).

One way of thinking about the session from a psychological point of view is to break it down into three five-minute chunks. Get through the first one and you've seen off a big part of the workload. Get through the second and you're into the final section. Once you're in the final section you're nearly there. Good luck!

Week 3 *Workout 1*

 Time **15 mins**   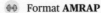 Format **AMRAP**

Exercise name	R1
1. Lunge arm raise	10
2. Offset press-up	6
3. Chair squat	12
4. Diagonal mountain climber	10
5. Crunch	10

Workout format and form guides

HOW TO DO IT
Do the reps for each of the five exercise in sequence to complete one round. Complete as many rounds as you can in 15 minutes. The pace you use and the rest periods that you take is down to you.

1. Lunge arm raise
Stand tall with your chest up, abs engaged and arms by your sides. Take a big step forwards with your left foot, then bend both knees to lunge down, while raising your arms directly overhead. Push through your front foot to return to the start, then step forwards with your right foot and repeat the move. Alternate your leading leg with each rep.

2. Offset press-up
Get on all fours with your legs and arms straight with your hands under your shoulders. Move your right hand out in front of you, then bend both elbows to lower your chest to the floor. Press back up to the start, then bring your right hand back underneath your shoulder. Move your left hand out in front of you and repeat.

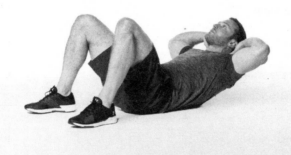

3. Chair squat
Stand tall with a chair behind you. Keeping your chest up and abs engaged, bend your knees to squat down and raise your arms in front of you to shoulder height. Once your glutes touch the chair, push through your heels to straighten your legs and stand back up to return to the start position.

4. Diagonal mountain climber
Get on all fours with your arms and legs straight. Without letting your hips sag, draw one knee in and bring it across towards the opposite elbow. Straighten that leg then repeat, bringing your other knee towards its opposite elbow Keep your abs engaged and the reps fast but controlled.

5. Crunch
Lie flat on your back with your knees bent and feet flat on the floor, and bend your arms so your fingers touch the side of your head. Engage your abs, then raise your torso off the floor without tensing your neck. Keep that tension on your abs as you slowly lower your torso back to the floor.

Week 3 *Workout 2*

 Time **15 mins**   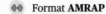 Format **AMRAP**

Exercise name	R1
1. Side lunge	10
2. Spider-man press-up	6
3. Overhead squat	12
4. Down-up	6
5. Reverse crunch	10

Workout format and form guides

HOW TO DO IT
Do the reps for each of the five exercise in sequence to complete one round. Complete as many rounds as you can in 15 minutes. The pace you use and the rest periods that you take is down to you.

1. Side lunge
Stand tall with your chest up, abs engaged and arms by your sides. Take a big step to your left, then bend your left leg to lunge down while raising your arms in front of you to shoulder height. Push through your left foot to return to the start, then repeat by taking a big step to your right. Alternate sides with each rep.

2. Spider-man press-up
Start in the press-up position. Engage your abs and bend your elbows to lower your chest towards the floor. As you do, bring one knee up so that it touches your arm. Press back up to straighten your arms and return to the start position. Repeat, bringing in the other knee, and alternate sides with each rep.

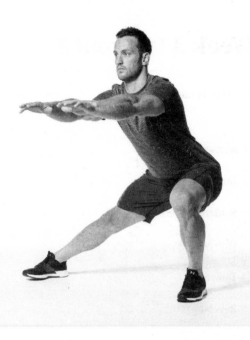

BONUS TIP: If you can't maintain good form, stop, take a few breaths, then resume the set. Repeat as much as needed.

3. Overhead squat
Stand tall with your chest up, abs engaged and arms raised directly overhead. Bend your knees to squat down as low as you can, keeping your arms straight overhead. Push through your heels to straighten your legs and return to the start position.

4. Down-up
Stand tall with your chest up and arms by your sides. Drop down so your palms are on the floor with your knees by your chest. Kick your legs out so your body forms a straight line from head to heels. Bring your knees back under your body, then stand back up.

5. Reverse crunch
Lie flat on your back with your arms flat on the floor and knees bent. Use your lower abs to draw your knees in towards your chest, then raise your hips up off the ground, then lower back to the start, keeping your abs fully engaged throughout.

Week 3 *Workout 3*

 Time **15 mins**   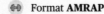 Format **AMRAP**

Exercise name	R1
1. Lunge with side bend	10
2. 1 and 1/4 press-up	6
3. Pulse squat	12
4. Burpee	6
5. Leg raise	10

Workout format and form guides

HOW TO DO IT
Do the reps for each of the five exercise in sequence to complete one round. **Complete as many rounds as you can in 15 minutes. The pace you use and the rest periods that you take is down to you.**

1. Lunge with side bend
Stand with your chest up, abs engaged and arms raised straight above your head. Take a big step forwards with your left foot and bend both knees to lunge while leaning over to your left. Push through your front foot to return to the start, then step forwards with your right foot and lean to your right. Alternate sides each rep.

2. 1 and 1/4 press-up
Get in the press-up position with your body in a straight line from head to heels. Engage your abs and bend your elbows to lower your chest towards the floor. Go as low as you can, then press back up one-quarter of the way then go back down to the bottom position. Press back up powerfully.

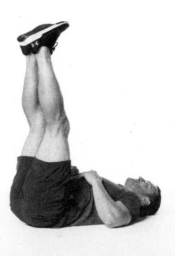

3. Pulse squat

Stand tall with your chest up, abs engaged and arms straight by your sides. Bend your knees to squat down as low as you can, either keeping your arms by your sides or raising them to shoulder height. In the bottom position of the squat, "pulse" up and down three times, then straighten your legs to return to the start position.

4. Burpee

Stand tall with your chest up and arms by your sides. Drop down so your palms are on the floor with your knees by your chest. Kick your legs out so your body forms a straight line from head to heels. Bring your knees back under your body, then jump up into the air. As you land, go straight into the next rep.

5. Leg raise

Lie flat on your back with your legs straight. Engage your abs, then raise your feet off the floor. Keeping your legs straight, raise your feet as high as you can, then slowly lower them. You can make the move harder and work your lower abs more by not allowing your heels to touch the floor between reps.

Week 3 *Workout 4*

⏱ Time **15 mins**   〽 Format **AMRAP**

Exercise name	R1
1. Bulgarian split squat (left)	8
2. T press-up	6
3. Bulgarian split squat (right)	8
4. Press-up burpee	8
5. Bicycle	12

Workout format and form guides

HOW TO DO IT
Do the reps for each of the five exercise in sequence to complete one round. Complete as many rounds as you can in 15 minutes. The pace you use and the rest periods that you take is down to you.

1. Bulgarian split squat (left)
Stand tall on your left leg with your right foot placed on a chair or raised surface behind you. Keeping your chest up and abs engaged, bend your left knee to lunge down as far as you can. Push back off your left foot to return to the start position and repeat.

2. T press-up
Get into the press-up position. Engage your abs and bend your elbows to lower your chest towards the floor. Go as low as you can, then press back up. As you do, rotate your torso to raise one arm straight up. Lower it and go straight into the next rep, turning the other way and raising your other arm. Alternate sides each rep.

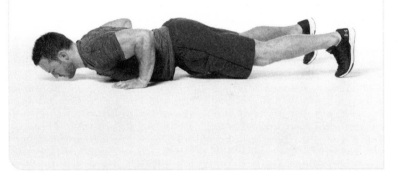

3. Bulgarian split squat (right)
Stand tall on your right leg with your left foot placed on a chair or raised surface behind you. Keeping your chest up and abs engaged, bend your right knee to lunge down as far as you can. Push back off your right foot to return to the start position and repeat.

4. Press-up burpee
Stand with your chest up and arms by your sides. Drop down so your palms are on the floor with your knees by your chest. Kick your legs out so your body forms a straight line from head to heels then perform a single press-up. Bring your knees back under your body, then jump up into the air. As you land, go straight into the next rep.

5. Bicycle
Lie on your back with your hands by your head and legs straight. Raise your torso and feet and engage your abs. Crunch up and rotate your torso to one side, bringing in your opposite knee to touch your elbow. Reverse the move back to the start, then repeat on the other side. Alternate sides each rep.

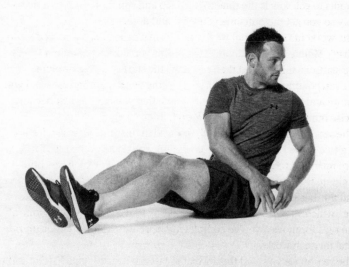

Week 4

You're into the final week of the plan, which means you only have three workouts to go! Now is the time to dig deep and summon every last ounce of energy so you get the outcome you want and deserve.

The workouts in this final week use a format called EMOM, which stands for Every Minute On the Minute. That means you do a set amount of work at the start of a minute and then rest until the start of the next minute when you continue with your workout. As the workout progresses and you get more and more tired, the length of time that you have to rest between exercise bursts reduces, making it even harder.

The sessions in this week are all arranged in the same way. You'll start with a two-move EMOM (exercise 1a and 1b). You do all of the reps for 1a before moving straight on to do all of the reps for 1b. You then rest until the minute is up and move on to the next EMOM (exercises 2a and 2b). The round finishes with a slightly more forgiving single move EMOM - an abs move - which should give you a bit more time to rest. Once you've done all of the reps for move 3 you've completed one round. There are four rounds in total for each workout.

The reason we've saved this format to last is because it gets harder as the session progresses and that's a tough thing to do from both a physical and a psychological point of view. Our advice is to just take it one round at a time and give it everything you've got. After all - at the end of this week you'll have completed the plan and that's the time for you to rest and recover.

Week 4 *Workout 1*

 Time **15 mins**   Format **EMOM**

Exercise name	R1	R2	R3	R4
1a. Lunge	12	10	8	6
1b. Decline press-up	10	8	6	4
2a. Squat	12	10	8	6
2b. Mountain climber	12	10	8	6
3. Crunch reach	12	10	8	6

Workout format and form guides

HOW TO DO IT
Start a stopwatch then do the round 1 reps of 1a then do the reps of 1b. Rest until 60 secs have elapsed then do the reps of 2a and the reps of 2b. Rest until 120 secs have elapsed then do the reps of 3. That's one round. Do four rounds, following the rep counts and resting 60 secs between rounds.

1a. Lunge
Stand with your chest up, abs engaged and arms by your sides. Take a big step forwards with your left foot, then bend both knees to lunge down until your right knee almost touches the floor. Push through your left foot to return to the start, then step forwards with your right foot and repeat the move, alternating leading legs each rep.

1b. Decline press-up
Get into the press-up position but with your feet on a box or raised platform. Your body should form a straight line from head to heels. Engage your abs and bend your elbows to lower your chest towards the floor. Go as low as you can, then press back up to straighten your arms and return to the start position.

GET FIT FAST AT HOME

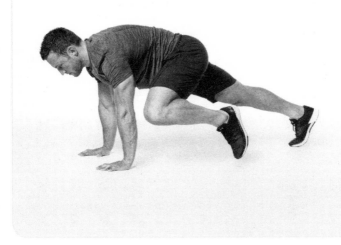

2a. Squat
Stand tall with your chest up, abs engaged and arms straight by your sides. Bend your knees and push your glutes backwards to squat down as low as you can, either keeping your arms by your sides or raising them up to shoulder height. Push through your heels to straighten your legs and return to the start position.

2b. Mountain climber
Get on all fours with your arms and legs straight and your wrists directly under your shoulders. Without letting your hips sag, draw one knee up and bring it towards the elbow on the same side. Straighten that leg, then repeat, bringing your other knee towards your elbow. Keep your abs engaged and keep the reps fast but controlled.

3. Crunch reach
Lie flat on your back with knees bent and arms straight and pointing up. Engage your abs to raise your torso up as high as you can, while reaching upwards towards the ceiling. Hold this top position for a second, then lower your torso back to the start. Make it harder by not allowing your upper back to touch the floor between reps.

Week 4 *Workout 2*

⏱ Time **15 mins**   ⟷ Format **EMOM**

Exercise name	R1	R2	R3	R4
1a. Reverse lunge	12	10	8	6
1b. Press-up	10	8	6	4
2a. Chair squat	12	10	8	6
2b. Jumping jacks	12	10	8	6
3. V-up	12	10	8	6

Workout format and form guides

HOW TO DO IT
Start a stopwatch then do the round 1 reps of 1a then do the reps of 1b. Rest until 60 secs have elapsed then do the reps of 2a and the reps of 2b. Rest until 120 secs have elapsed then do the reps of 3. That's one round. Do four rounds, following the rep counts and resting 60 secs between rounds.

1a. Reverse lunge
Stand tall with your chest up, abs engaged and arms by your sides. Take a big step backwards with your left foot, then bend both knees to lunge down. Push through your back foot to return to the start, then step backwards with your right foot and repeat the move. Alternate sides with each rep.

1b. Press-up
Get into the press-up position with your legs and arms straight, and your hands under your shoulders. Your body should form a straight line from head to heels. Engage your abs and bend your elbows to lower your chest towards the floor. Go as low as you can, then press up to straighten your arms and return to the start.

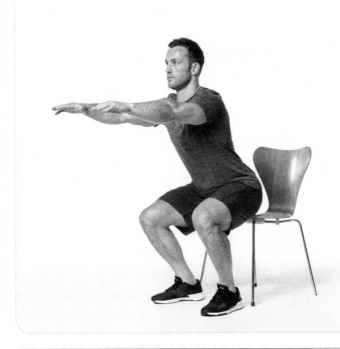

BONUS TIP: It can be tempting to rush your reps, but for the best results ensure your muscles - not momentum - do all of the work.

2A. Chair squat
Stand tall with a chair behind you. Keeping your chest up and abs engaged, bend your knees to squat down and raise your arms in front of you to shoulder height. Once your glutes touch the chair, push through your heels to straighten your legs and stand back up to return to the start position.

2B. Jumping jacks
Stand tall with your chest up, abs engaged and hands by your sides. Jump up and bring both feet out wide to the sides while raising your arms to the sides so your hands finish above your head. Jump back from the wide stance to the start position, lowering your arms as you go.

3. V-up
Lie flat on your back with your legs straight and your arms straight pointing behind you. Engage your abs and with your arms and legs straight, raise your arms and feet off the floor, and bring your arms forwards so your hands touch your legs. Reverse the movement to return to the start.

Week 4 *Workout 3*

 Time **15 mins**   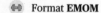 Format **EMOM**

Exercise name	R1	R2	R3	R4
1a. Lunge reach	12	10	8	6
1b. Incline press-up	10	8	6	4
2a. Overhead squat	12	10	8	6
2b. Diagonal mountain climber	12	10	8	6
3. Russian twist	12	10	8	6

Workout format and form guides

HOW TO DO IT
Start a stopwatch then do the round 1 reps of 1a then do the reps of 1b. Rest until 60 secs have elapsed then do the reps of 2a and the reps of 2b. Rest until 120 secs have elapsed then do the reps of 3. That's one round. Do four rounds, following the rep counts and resting 60 secs between rounds.

1a. Lunge reach
Stand with your chest up, abs engaged and arms straight above your head. Take a big step forwards with your left foot and bend both knees to lunge down while leaning over to your left. Push through your front foot to return to the start, then step forwards with your right foot and repeat the move, leaning to your right. Alternate sides each rep.

1b. Incline press-up
Start in the press-up position but with your hands under your shoulders on a box or raised platform. Your body should form a straight line from head to heels. Engage your abs and bend your elbows to lower your chest towards the floor. Go as low as you can, then press back up to straighten your arms and return to the start position.

BONUS TIP: Don't lie on the floor in your rest periods between rounds - use it to do some light stretching or mobility moves.

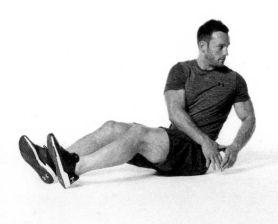

2a. Overhead squat
Stand tall with your chest up, abs engaged and arms raised directly overhead. Bend your knees to squat down as low as you can, keeping your arms straight overhead. Push through your heels to straighten your legs and return to the start position.

2b. Diagonal mountain climber
Get on all fours with your arms and legs straight. Without letting your hips sag, draw one knee in and bring it across towards the opposite elbow. Straighten that leg then repeat, bringing your other knee towards its opposite elbow Keep your abs engaged and the reps fast but controlled.

5. Russian twist
Sit up with your chest up, abs engaged and a slight bend in your knees. Use your abs to rotate your torso to one side, then return to the middle and rotate to the other side. Make the move harder by raising your heels off the floor and keeping them raised.

Week 4 *Workout 4*

⏱ Time **15 mins**   🏋 Format **EMOM**

Exercise name	R1	R2	R3	R4
1a. Side lunge	12	10	8	6
1b. Spider-man press-up	10	8	6	4
2a. 1 and 1/4 squat	12	10	8	6
2b. Burpee	12	10	8	6
3. Thread the needle	12	10	8	6

Workout format and form guides

HOW TO DO IT
Start a stopwatch then do the round 1 reps of 1a then do the reps of 1b. Rest until 60 secs have elapsed then do the reps of 2a and the reps of 2b. Rest until 120 secs have elapsed then do the reps of 3. That's one round. Do four rounds, following the rep counts and resting 60 secs between rounds.

1a. Side lunge
Stand tall with your chest up, abs engaged and arms by your sides. Take a big step to your left, then bend your left leg to lunge down while raising your arms in front of you to shoulder height. Push through your left foot to return to the start, then repeat by taking a big step to your right. Alternate sides with each rep.

1b. Spider-man press-up
Start in the press-up position. Engage your abs and bend your elbows to lower your chest towards the floor. As you do, bring one knee up so that it touches your arm. Press back up to straighten your arms and return to the start position. Repeat, bringing in the other knee, and alternate sides with each rep.

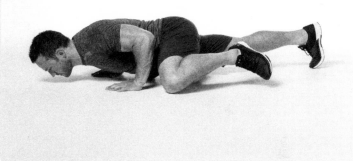

2a. 1 and 1/4 squat
Stand with your chest up, abs engaged and arms straight by your sides. Bend your knees to squat down as low as you can, either keeping your arms by your sides or raising them to shoulder height. From the bottom position of the squat, come back up one-quarter of the way to standing back up, then squat down before then standing up.

2b. Burpee
Stand tall with your chest up and arms by your sides. Drop down so your palms are on the floor with your knees by your chest. Kick your legs out so your body forms a straight line from head to heels. Bring your knees back under your body, then jump up into the air. As you land, go straight into the next rep.

3. Thread the needle
Get into position, supporting yourself on your forearms with your elbows underneath your shoulders. Lift one hand off the floor. Rotate your torso and raise that arm. Rotate back down and move that arm underneath your body, then rotate back again. Do half the stated number of reps, then switch sides and do the other half.

Part 3
Progression

Take your health and fitness to the next level

Congratulations! You've completed your 28-day training programme, and you will now be looking and feeling better than ever. And while it's important to celebrate your achievements and take pride in the progress you've made over the past month, in many ways now is the perfect time to think about how you can build upon the impressive foundations you've just laid, and what you want to achieve next, so that you can continue to take your health and fitness onwwards and upwards to the next level.

One easy option is to repeat the 28-day plan that you've just completed and see if you can beat your rep counts from the first time you did it. You can do that because it will still provide enough of a challenge to your mind and muscles. Of course, if you keep doing the same thing over and over again, you'll get bored and your progress will stall so you will need to do new things. This chapter will explain how you can take the next steps on your journey towards your best-ever body - all in the comfort of your own home. So keep reading to get up to speed with the latest tried-and-tested home workout tips, advice and insight so you can continue to make rapid progress by burning fat effectively, building new lean muscle mass quickly, improving your cardiovascular fitness, and build on your new strength to keep getting stronger and achieve real-world strength and fitness.

Create your own HIIT workouts

Do HIIT at home to burn fat and build muscle

As you now know from first-hand experience, high-intensity interval training is a fantastic weapon in your fat-burning arsenal, as well as being extremely helpful in building muscle mass and improving cardiovascular fitness. And one of the very best things about HIIT is that a workout can take hundreds of different forms - the only real limit is your imagination! You can use your own bodyweight to do press-ups, squats and lunges for an anytime-anywhere HIIT session, or use kettlebells, barbells or dumbbells, or any combination of the above, for a calorie-burning, heart-raising workout. Whatever equipment you prefer, here are the key considerations that should underpin every successful HIIT session.

WORKOUT LENGTH

The very nature of HIIT workouts - that your effort level should be very intense and close to your maximum capacity - means that sessions are always short: they can't be long because it's impossible to sustain all-out effort for any serious length of time. If you think you can do a HIIT session non-stop for more than 20 or 30 minutes that doesn't mean you're super-fit; it proves you're not actually training at a particularly intense level. Indeed, some HIIT protocols last only four minutes: the Tabata approach of 20 seconds of maximum effort intensity, interspersed with 10 seconds of rest, repeated eight times, is one of the shortest yet most effective exercise strategies to improve cardiovascular fitness. While quality of training is more important that quantity of time spent training, aim at first to do HIIT sessions in 10 to 20 minutes, with between 50%-75% of the time "working" and the rest "resting". The longer the session, the closer the ratio between work and rest.

EXERCISE SELECTION

The moves you do are entirely down to the kit you have available and your own personal preferences. For example, if you are short

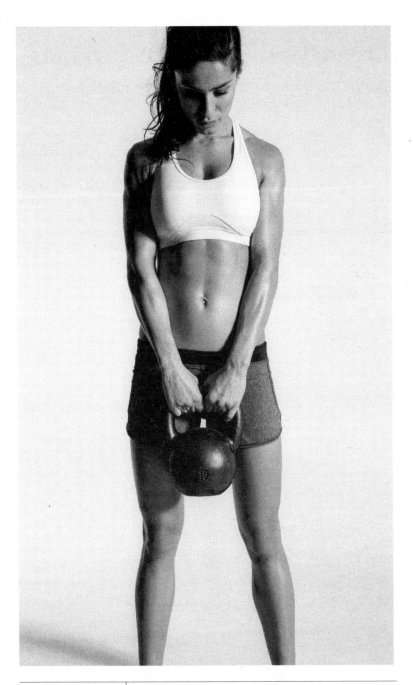

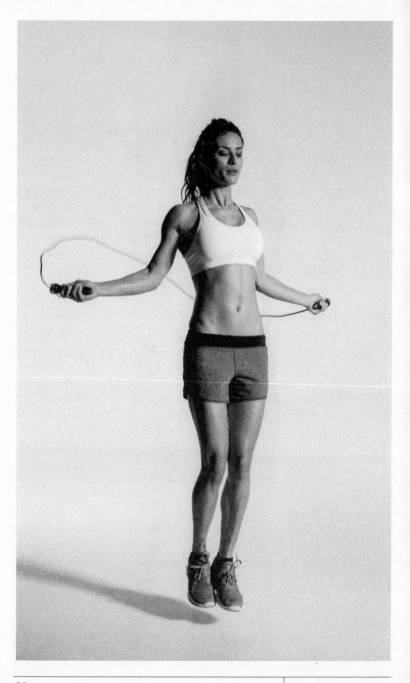

of time and kit you can do a very simple HIIT session, such as 10
burpees every minute on the minute for 10 minutes: that will get
your heart-rate up and a good sweat on. If you have dumbbells
you can construct a full-body HIIT session - think 10 squats into 10
lunges into 10 shoulder presses into 10 press-ups into 10 dumbbell
rows into 10 crunches - that will work every major muscle group
to burn fat and build muscle. The most important factor behind a
successful HIIT session is ultimately compliance: you'll only reap
the benefits if you do it, so it makes sense to design a session or
sessions that move you towards you number one fitness goal as
well as ones that you'll look forward to doing.

WORK-TO-REST PROTOCOLS
As mentioned above, the shorter your session the more time you
can spend working versus resting. That's because you can push
yourself harder in a shorter session - if you're doing a five-minute
blast you could do 40-seconds on, 20-seconds off and keep your
intensity levels high - whereas a 20-minute session will require
more substantial rest periods to give yourself time to recover
before your next all-out work set. One strategy would be to start
with a 50-50 work-to-rest ratio, then adjust it up and down based
on how you feel, and gradually increase the work periods whilst
reducing the rest periods as your fitness levels improve.

WORKOUT FREQUENCY
HIIT sessions are very hard - it's why they're so effective. As well
as taxing your heart, lungs and muscles in a short amount of time,
they also fatigue your central nervous system (CNS): intense work
requires faster muscle contractions and that tires your CNS faster
than normal cardio. At first leave at least a day between HIIT
workouts, especially if they're similar in exercise selection and
structure. As you become more experienced you can do different
HIIT sessions on concurrent days to get all the benefits without
overloading your CNS or muscles.

Key home gym kit

Torch fat and build muscle with basic kit

The beauty of high-intensity home workouts is that you don't need any specialist equipment to start a session: your own bodyweight provides ample resistance to work most of your major muscle groups, like squats to work your glutes and legs, and press-ups to hit your chest, shoulders and triceps. But if you do have access to some very simple weight-training kit, such as a pair of adjustable dumbbells or a kettlebell, you have everything you need to work all your major muscles to not only improve your cardiovascular fitness and burn fat, but also to add lean muscular size to your frame.

Many people will have a set of dumbbells (most likely in the garage, under the bed, or as a make-shift door stop), but even if you don't you can pick up a basic pair very cheaply online. The same goes for a kettlebell: all you need is one to add some extra resistance to your HIIT workouts to challenge your heart, lungs and muscles in new ways to elicit ever-greater fat-loss and muscle-building results. Here's what you need to know.

Training with dumbbells

Are they a good home gym option?
Yes. Dumbbells are one of the most versatile bits of weight-lifting kit because you can target every single muscle group with them. A basic set is cheap but worth its weight in gold if you want to get leaner and stronger. They're also good value for money and they don't take up much space. If you only buy one piece of home workout kit, this is a great option.

What kind of fitness do they build?
With dumbbells you can improve cardiovascular fitness, burn body fat and build lean muscle mass. Crucially, you can do compound moves, which work multiple muscle groups at once and isolation exercises, which directly target individual muscles.

What's a good entry level product?
An adjustable set so you can change how heavy they are for different moves. You want to get a set that gives you the option to lift at least 10kg each side. Heavier sets will make it easier to challenge the stronger muscle groups in your body, such as your quads and hamstrings. You can get sets that make it incredibly quick to adjust the weight, but they can be quite expensive.

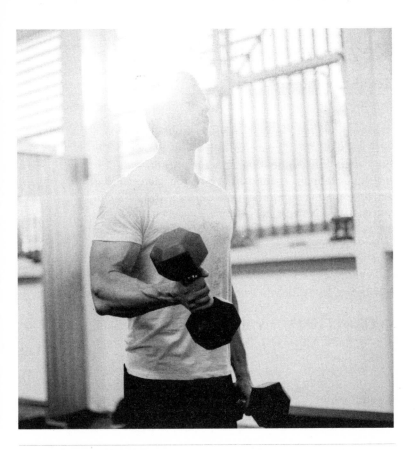

Training with kettlebells

Are they a good home gym option?
They are an excellent home gym
option because you can do so many
exercises and types of workout with
just one kettlebell. The main difference
between kettlebells and dumbbells is
that the former require a higher level
of technical ability due to the very
dynamic nature of the exercises.

What kind of fitness do they build?
They've very versatile items of kit.
They're excellent at developing
explosive power, because moves such
as swings and snatches are fast and
dynamic exercises. You can also use
them to develop your cardio fitness
and for fat loss. They're not brilliant
for isolation work but that's probably
not the most important element of a
home workout, and the amount of big
compound moves you can do will help
to build an impressive physique and
level of strength and fitness.

What's a good entry level product?
A 12kg or 16kg kettlebell is a good
entry-level product. That may sound
quite heavy but because you generally
perform big compound moves rather
than isolation exercises, it's an
appropriate place to start.

Part 4
Nutrition

Eat right to fuel your workouts and accelerate fat loss

What's more important when you're trying to get in shape - diet or exercise? The truth is that they are both important and the smartest and most sensible approaches to health and fitness take both into account. After all, what's the point of putting your time and effort into a training session only to undo it by scoffing a bag of doughnuts afterwards? Equally, how fit do you think you'll get by chomping carrots while sitting on your sofa?

If you want to maximise your results you need to be aware of what you eat. The good news is that's probably easier and more enjoyable than you might imagine. You don't have to eat 'perfectly' (not that that word means much when it comes to nutrition) all the time but you do need to consume a wide range of fresh food.

This section gives you the information you need to make smart and sustainable food choices, because the best way of eating is the one you can sustain over time. If a nutrition approach has good results in the short term but is so restrictive and unappealing that you can't sustain it for more than a few weeks then it's not a great approach. Food should always be something you enjoy and something that can be sociable, rather than something you associate with restriction and denial. So read the advice over the following pages to make sure it's body fat, and not flavour, that you get rid of.

Calorie condundrum

The final word on whether calories matter

Calories are probably the most hotly-contested subject in the world of nutrition and healthy eating. The two big camps at oppposing ends of the debate are those who think that calories are the only thing that matters, and then those who think that counting calories is a complete waste of time.

Well, neither of those extreme views are helpful, but there's a bit of sense on both sides if you dig deep enough and we'll go into why in more detail below. One of the things that you should be aware of is that there are psychological elements to calories, as well as the literal numbers that they represent. Food can be a hugely emotional subject, so forcing someone to obsess over numbers, and then to make them feel guilty because they consumed 50 calories more in a meal than they were supposed to isn't a healthy approach. The broad approach we'd advocate is to be aware of the calorie content of your food, but not to be obsessed by it.

Calorie quantity

The main reason why people think that counting calories is important is because, fundamentally, you need to burn more calories than you consume if you want to lose fat. That's because excess calories will ultimately be stored as body fat. Conversely, if you are in a calorie deficit your body will use some of its fat stores as fuel. This is the main reason why it makes sense to be aware of the rough amount of calories you're consuming.

If you do want to lose body fat then we'd suggest that you aim to be in a small but sustainable daily calorie deficit of about 200 calories.

There's no perfect figure. The point is that you don't want or need a huge calorie deficit. If, for example, you are in a daily deficit of about 1,000 calories then you will lose weight but you'll feel hungry and tired, which isn't much fun. You may also be catabolising (burning) muscle tissue because your body is so desperate for fuel. And you may be missing out on vital nutrients that are crucial for many biological functions. So think small and sustainable and you're on the right lines. You also don't need to be absolutely precise because that approach can become obsessive.

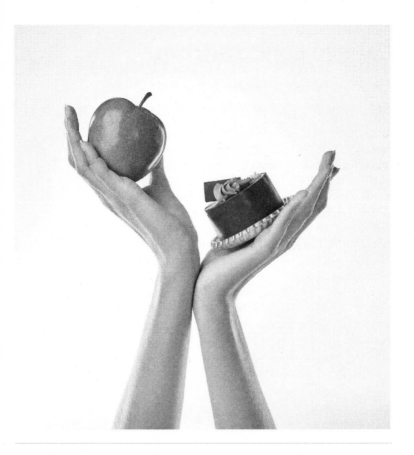

Calorie quality

If losing weight is all about being in a small but sustainable calorie deficit then that's all you've got to worry about, right? Well, it's not quite that simple, because it's not just how much you eat that matters. What you eat is also important. For example, all food is made up of three main macronutrients - protein, carbohydrates and fats - and that's what determines its calorie content. But food is also made up of micronutrients - the vitamins and minerals that are responsible for a broad range of biological functions in your body. If you don't get a sufficient quantity of these vitamins and minerals your health might suffer.

The easiest way of ensuring that you are getting the right nutrients is to eat a wide variety of fresh food and to avoid cutting out any major food groups, unless you have a specific intolerance or allergy. So a diet that's rich in meat, fish, eggs, dairy, vegetables, fruit, nuts, seeds and grains will give you a balanced diet. You'll also find that this kind of nutritionally-dense food will make you feel full for longer so you'll be less inclined to overeat, which will further assist your fat-loss efforts.

How many calories do you need?

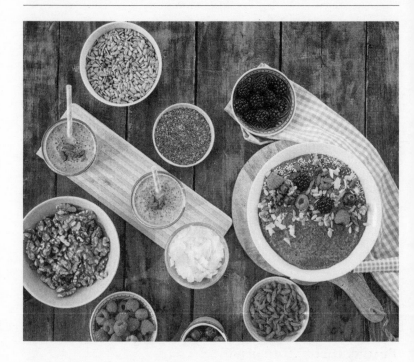

As we established on the previous page, it is useful to know how many calories you're consuming for one simple reason: eat fewer calories than you burn and you lose weight; eat more calories than you burn and you gain weight. It's called the Energy Balance Equation and here it is:

Change in body stores = Energy In – Energy Out

The equation says "body stores" rather than "bodyweight" because body stores refers to the bodily tissues, such as muscle and fat, that are affected by a positive or negative energy balance equation. "Bodyweight" can be significantly impacted by changes in body water, but those changes are only temporary and have nothing to do with your body-fat levels.

Calculating your energy needs

Accurately assessing your daily energy requirements can be complex, requiring you to input your height, weight, age, gender, activity levels, goals and other data into mathematical equations.

Thankfuly there's an easier way - use the chart below. It gets you as close as you need to be to the same daily calorie number in a fraction of the time. The formula is in pounds (lb) - there are 14lb in one stone. In general women should use the smaller multipliers in each box and men the larger one. If you know your weight in kilos, multiply it by 2.2 to convert it to pounds.

Your activity level	YOUR GOAL		
	Lose Fat	Maintain Weight	Gain Muscle
Lightly Active (<3 hrs/wk)	Bodyweight (lb) x 10-12	Bodyweight (lb) x 12-14	Bodyweight (lb) x 16-18
Moderately Active (3-6 hrs/wk)	Bodyweight (lb) x 12-14	Bodyweight (lb) x 14-16	Bodyweight (lb) x 18-20
Very Active (>6 hrs/wk)	Bodyweight (lb) x 14-16	Bodyweight (lb) x 16-18	Bodyweight (lb) x 20-22

Putting theory into practice

To understand how the numbers work in real life, here are two examples:

EXAMPLE 1
A 160lb (11st 6lb), moderately active woman wanting to lose fat
She would estimate her calorie needs by multiplying her weight in pounds x 12, which is 160 x 12 = 1,920.
To lose weight she would require approximately 1,920 calories daily.

EXAMPLE 2
A 190lb (13st 8lb), moderately active man wanting to gain muscle
He would estimate his calorie needs by multiplying his weight in pounds x 20, which is 190 x 20 = 3,800.
To gain weight he would require approximately 3,800 calories daily.

Macros made simple

Here's a guide to the components in the food you eat

As we established earlier in the chapter, food is made up of three main macronutrients - proteins, carbohydrates and fats. Understanding the basics behind these macronutrients will help you to create a balanced and sustainable diet. Here's what you need to know.

What are macronutrients?
Macronutrients are the three main groups of chemical compounds that make up the food we eat. They are protein, fats and carbohydrates.

What are micronutrients?
Micronutrients are chemical compounds such as vitamins, minerals and phytonutrients (plant-based nutrients) in food. They are found in much smaller quantities than macronutrients, and we only need them in very small amounts.

Macronutrients

Protein
After water, most of what makes you, well, you is made from proteins, and all proteins are made from amino acids. There are many types of amino acid, most of which your body can manufacture itself when required, but there are nine amino acids your body can't synthesise. They're called "essential amino acids" and you must get them from food. Most foods contain at least small (or "trace") amounts of protein, but these are some of the most protein-rich foods.

Animal sources
- Poultry (chicken, turkey, duck, goose) and eggs
- Red meat (beef, pork, lamb)
- Wild game (venison, rabbit, pheasant)
- Fish and shellfish
- Dairy (milk, cheese, yogurt)

Plant sources
- Beans and legumes
- Tofu, tempeh and other soy products
- Nuts and seeds (though these are generally much higher in fat than protein)
- Some grains such as quinoa, amaranth and wild rice (though these are much higher in carbohydrates than protein)

How much do I need?

A good target is about 0.8g-1g of protein per kilogram of bodyweight per day, but you may need more if you're very active, older, pregnant or breastfeeding, or ill or injured.

Carbohydrates

There are many types of carbohydrates and they're mainly found in plant-based foods. Some carbs are very simple molecules, such as sugars, which are the most basic form. Others are much more complicated and are called complex carbohydrates. Starches, which are found in potatoes and beans, are one type of complex carb, as is fibre.

The more "simple" the carbohydrate the easier it is to digest and absorb. In general, when eating for better health and fitness you want to prioritise consuming complex carbohydrates because they are slower-digesting and more nutrient-rich than simple carbs.

Our bodies can't completely break down some types of complex carbs, such as insoluble fibre or resistant starch, but the bacteria in our gut love it and make other beneficial compounds from it. Fibre and resistant starch are often known as "prebiotics": they're food sources that nourish our "good" gut bacteria. Fibre also helps move things through our intestinal tract.

Higher-fibre foods include fruits and vegetables, whole grains, beans and legumes, and nuts and seeds, and resistant starch is found in beans, green bananas, and many other plant-based foods.

Best sources of fibre and micronutrient-rich carbs
- Sweet and starchy vegetables (winter squashes, beetroot)

- Starchy tubers (potatoes, sweet potatoes, yams)
- Whole grains (rice, wheat, oats)
- Beans and legumes
- Fruit

How much do I need?

That depends on myriad factors, including your activity levels: you need more carbs if you are physically active and/or trying to build muscle. While some people do benefit from a lower-carb diet, most people look, feel and perform better from eating at least some carbs, especially the nutrient-rich, higher-fibre types.

Fats

The main three types of dietary fat are saturated, monounsaturated and polyunsaturated (see below). They differ from one another by the number and frequency of the carbon atoms that bond them, but you don't need to worry about that. You just need to know that fats are an essential macronutrient and you need to consume them for optimal health (it's yet another reason why very low-fat "detox diets" make you look and feel so bad).

The three types of healthy fat

Most fat sources contain more than one type of dietary fat, but these foods are particularly high in one type

Saturated
- Butter and high-fat dairy (eg cheese)
- Most animal fats
- Coconut and coconut oil
- Egg yolk
- Cacao butter

Monounsaturated
- Avocado
- Olives and olive oil
- Peanuts
- Many types of nuts, such as pecans and almonds

Polyunsaturated
- Many types of seeds such as flax, chia, sesame and sunflower seeds
- Oily fish such as salmon, herring, and mackerel

How much do I need?

Most people do best with 25-35% of their total daily calories coming from a wide variety of healthy fat sources. Omega-3 fatty acids, particularly EPA and DHA, are special types of fats found in oily fish, seafood and some plant sources. They can help you lose weight, boost brain function, reduce inflammation, and improve both your physical and mental health – they're all-round performers.

You may have noticed that processed cooking oils, margarine and cooking sprays don't appear here and with good reason. Most "long life" cooking oils and margarines are heavily processed and contain types of fat called "trans fats" that aren't found in nature, so your body doesn't know how to process them. Research increasingly suggests trans fats contribute to many health problems.

Micronutrients

Vitamins and minerals come in many forms and what we think of as a "vitamin" or a "mineral" is actually a group of molecules that are chemically similar, but sufficiently different to do different jobs in the body. For example "vitamin A" is actually a family of molecules, and the carotenoid forms of vitamin A (such as beta-carotene) are water-soluble, found mainly in plants (such as carrots), and not very well absorbed; while the retinoid forms of vitamin A are fat-soluble, found mostly in animal foods (such as egg yolks) and are well absorbed.

We absorb minerals such as calcium, iron and magnesium from dairy and meat better than from leafy greens, which come in harder-to-digest forms. This is one reason why it's important to eat a wide variety of foods: each food has a unique chemical "fingerprint" of micronutrients that contributes to our good health.

You may think taking a multi-vitamin or multi-mineral supplement helps you avoid deficiencies, but taking more vitamin and/or mineral pills is not usually better or healthier. Instead, focus on improving the quality and variety of your food choices so that you get your vitamins and minerals in the form that nature intended.

Fat loss food rules

Take these ideas on board to keep your diet on track

LIMIT PROCESSED FOOD

The reason we're advising you to do this is because processed food tends to be low in nutrients, easy to overeat and high in unhelpful things like sugar and trans fats. We're not saying that you can never eat this kind of food, or that you can never eat refined sugar or trans fats but you should generally aim to limit their consumption.

COOK FROM SCRATCH

One of the easiest ways to ensure that you limit your processed food consumption is to cook your meals yourself, rather than buying take aways or ready meals. Now, we appreciate that this can increase the amount of time you spend preparing food but healthy food doesn't have to take ages to cook. Grilling some seasoned chicken or fish with some chopped veg and serving it with some brown rice will only take about ten minutes.

EAT ENOUGH PROTEIN

If you'd like to improve your body composition (reduce fat levels while simultaneously adding lean muscle mass) then consuming adequate levels of protein will help you to do that. You don't need to be eating endless chicken breasts. You just need about 1.0-1.5g of protein per kilo of bodyweight per day. If you have a good protein serving with each main meal (eggs for breakfast, chicken salad for lunch and fish or meat at dinner, for example) you'll pretty much hit your target without thinking about it.

LOAD UP ON VEG

It's almost impossible to overeat vegetables. Partly because they are very low in calories, so you'd need to consume a vast quantity to tip yourself into a calorie excess. They are also high in nutrients such as fibre, which helps you to feel full. So don't think that you can only have one vegetable with a meal. There's no reason why you can't eat three or four in one meal. You could grill onions, peppers and courgettes with chicken, for example, and also serve that with some steamed green veg. Making salads is also a really easy way to increase your intake of veg.

FILL IN WITH CARBS

A simple but effective approach is to prioritise protein in your meals, then make sure you have a decent serving of healthy fats and then fill in the rest of your calorie count with carbohydrates. You can also choose your carb sources wisely. Go for brown rice and pasta rather than refined white options, which have been stripped of most of their nutrients. We should also point out that there is no need whatsoever to cut out all carbs.

CHEW YOUR FOOD

We're pretty sure that you've heard this one before but it really makes a difference. Firstly, you break your food down into smaller pieces, which helps you to use the nutrients in what you're eating while also aiding digestion. It will also give your brain time to register when you're full before you've overeaten.

DON'T EAT DISTRACTED

Another good habit to get into for mealtimes is to eat at a table, rather than in front of a screen. Studies have shown that eating in a distracted state can cause you to eat more. So eat your meals at a table, slow down and enjoy them.

DON'T GO HUNGRY

A big mistake a lot of people make when they try to get fit is to drastically reduce the quantity of food they eat. But if you do this to the extent that you are ravenous then the chances are that when you do come to eat you'll be craving really calorie-dense foods. It's a lot easier to make healthy food choices when your stomach isn't grumbling and your brain isn't begging you to gobble up a massive pie.

Fat loss foods

Add these foods to your diet to get lean fast

In order to make healthy eating a bit easier, we've compiled a list of some of our favourite foods that you can be sure will help you achieve your better-body goals. It's not an exhaustive list but it gives you an idea of the kinds of foods that are high in the kind of nutrients that you're looking for. There are also plenty of great foods that aren't on the list so use it as a starting point and add in any kind of meat, fish, fruit, veg, nuts and seeds that you like. It's also worth pointing out that other foods, such as chocolates, aren't completely off-limits. Our advice is just to limit those types of treats and snacks and focus on fresh foods.

Food (100g unless stated)	Cals	Protein	Carbs	Fat
Meat and fish				
Chicken breast	120	27g	0g	1g
Turkey breast	117	24g	0g	2g
Lean sirloin steak	176	26g	0g	7g
Lean beef mince	124	21g	0g	5g
Lamb	136	22g	0g	5g
Lean pork chops	184	32g	0g	6g
Honey roast ham	120	20g	1g	4g
Roast beef	136	24g	1g	4g
Salmon fillet	190	21g	0g	12g

Food	Cals	Protein	Carbs	Fats
Smoked salmon	179	21g	0g	14g
White fish	93	21g	0g	1g
Prawns	72	16g	0g	1g
Tuna steak	105	24g	0g	1g
Eggs and dairy				
Eggs	143	13g	1g	10g
Cheddar cheese	331	29g	0g	24g
Low-fat Greek yogurt	75	6g	7g	3g
Butter	730	0g	0g	81g
Semi-skimmed milk	50	3g	5g	2g
Grains and carbs				
Wholemeal bread	224	9g	42g	2g
Brown rice	353	8g	77g	1g
Potatoes	75	2g	18g	0g
Wholemeal pasta	353	11g	72g	2g
Vermicelli noodles	353	7g	79g	1g

Food	Cals	Protein	Carbs	Fats
Healthy fats				
Avocado	190	2g	2g	20g
Rapeseed oil	864	0g	0g	96g
Low-fat mayo	300	1g	9g	29g
Peanut butter	623	23g	13g	54g
Brazil nuts (20g)	136	3g	0g	14g
Coconut milk	186	1g	5g	18g
Pine nuts	695	16g	4g	68g
Fruit				
Apples	48	0g	12g	0g
Bananas	90	1g	21g	0g
Blueberries	56	0g	14g	0g
Strawberries	28	1g	6g	0g
Oranges	40	1g	9g	0g
Grapefruit	28	1g	7g	0g
Grapes	64	1g	15g	0g

Food	Cals	Protein	Carbs	Fats
Vegetables				
Carrots	32	1g	7g	0g
Onion	38	1g	8g	0g
Broccoli	33	4g	2g	1g
Tomato	16	1g	3g	0g
Mushroom	12	2g	1g	0g
Green beans	20	2g	3g	0g
Sugar snap peas	32	3g	5g	0g
Pepper	12	1g	2g	0g
Spinach	25	2g	2g	1g
Cucumber	12	1g	2g	0g
Courgette	16	2g	2g	0g
Celery	8	1g	1g	0g
Peas	73	6g	10g	1g
Red cabbage	20	1g	4g	0g

Water and other drinks

Make sure you're drinking enough to stay healthy

You've probably heard you need to drink eight glasses of water per day, but there's no hard evidence to support that. There are, however, some very good reasons to stay hydrated, particularly if you're aiming to lose weight. You see, dehydration is often mistaken for hunger, which may encourage you to eat when all you actually need is a glass of water.

There are simple ways to avoid dehydration: drink a big glass of water as soon as you wake up; pay more attention to thirst; drink more during exercise or in hot or humid conditions; choose water as your go-to drink (instead of alcohol or caffeinated drinks); and check your urine colour (the darker it is, the more dehydrated you are). If you often forget to drink enough water – you may notice you feel mentally and physically tired – fill up a water bottle at the beginning of the day, keep it close and take a big gulp every time you look at it.

LIQUID CALORIES

While we're advising you to drink more water, we're probably advising you to drink less of other drinks, particularly high-sugar ones such as fizzy drinks. We'd also suggest that you limit your consumption of fruit juice too. It's much better to eat the real thing. The reason we're making these suggestions is because it's easy to consume hundreds of calories from sugary drinks without realising it.

Different types of the same drink can also have a wildly different nutritional composition: a black coffee only contains about 5 calories, whereas a large latte can contain about 250.

LAST ORDERS

When it comes to alcohol, the less you consume the better - if fat loss is your aim. That doesn't mean you can never have a drink. You just need to be aware that a pint of beer will add about 200 calories to your daily total but hardly any useful nutrients. If you are going to drink, options such as a red wine or a clear spirit and low-calorie mixer are your best bet. The other thing to consider regarding alcohol is the extra food calories you generally consume during and after drinking. Oh, and the impact it has on your wallet, mood and sleep. Cheers!

Smart supplementation

Your instant guide to the most popular supplements

Supplements aren't magic pills - they won't give you a great body without you doing the work. And they shouldn't replace a balanced and healthy diet. They can, however, have a positive impact on your health and body composition, if you use the ones with most credible scientific research.

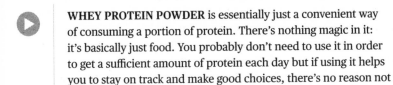

WHEY PROTEIN POWDER is essentially just a convenient way of consuming a portion of protein. There's nothing magic in it: it's basically just food. You probably don't need to use it in order to get a sufficient amount of protein each day but if using it helps you to stay on track and make good choices, there's no reason not to use it.

VITAMIN D3 plays an essential role in a huge number of biological and metabolic functions, as well as improving cognition, and reducing the risk of certain cancers, cardiovascular disease and dementia. You get it through exposure to sunlight but if you live in a country where you don't see much sun, you could use a supplement. Be aware that taking high doses can be toxic, because your body won't flush out excess levels. It can also deplete levels of other essential nutrients, such as vitamin K.

OMEGA-3 is an "essential" fatty acid, which means we need to consume it directly from our diet. Good sources of omega-3 include oily fish, nuts and seeds. Even though omega-3 is a fatty acid, it has been shown to have a positive impact on fat loss as well as positively impacting brain function, inflammation levels and cardiovascular health.

MULTIVITAMINS are probably one of the most commonly consumed supplements. Ideally you won't need to take one, because if you're eating a wide variety of fresh food then you won't need it. It can, however, be used as a "nutritional safety net" to ensure that if there are any gaps in your diet then you have them covered.

Part 5
Life

The benefits of balance for building a better body

In the pursuit of building a leaner, bigger or stronger body, it can be tempting to believe that the harder you go - so the more sessions you do per week, or the fewer carbs you eat each day - the faster you'll get the results you crave. The reality, however, is that building a better body requires a smart approach. Not just a smart approach to training (in making sure each workout is taking you closer to your goal), but also a smart approach to eating, recovery and living the rest of your life! A concerted effort to have a "balanced" lifestyle is crucial to achieving your best-ever body, as well as thriving and enjoying every single area of your existence. After all, what's the point of achieving Herculean strength if you spend every minute of every day plotting and planning your workouts, or measuring every single morsel that enters your mouth - and are utterly miserable as a result? Life is too short for that, so here's how to achieve that desirable balanced approach.

ENJOY THE RIDE
While your workouts should be tough, one of the best ways to know if you're doing too much too often is when training because a real chore that you dread. If that happens take a step back and re-appraise your approaches.

Recovery and journaling

Use these secret weapons to make faster progress

THE IMPORTANCE OF RECOVERY
Recovery is one of key aspects of improving your fitness that many people neglect to take seriously. But think of it this way: it's only during quality rest and recuperation periods that your body has the time and resources to rebuild your muscles bigger and stronger. In fact, if you train too hard too often and don't eat enough quality food, you'll shock your body into thinking you're in a dire situation. You'll no longer see positive results and will start to get weaker and stop losing fat because your body will prioritise using muscle tissue for fuel and preserve its fat stores for the perceived "crisis". Therefore, only do an intense workout every other day - never on consecutive days - eat enough high-quality protein, get a good 7-9 hours of sleep a night, and try to spend half an hour each day on a non-exercise activity you enjoy.

COMPLEMENT YOUR HIIT WITH LISS
Though you shouldn't do intense workouts on consecutive days, you can use your regular "rest" days to do other types of exercise, such as active recovery sessions (think Pilates, yoga, walking or stretching) or LISS (low-intensity steady state) workouts, such as jogging, cycling or swimming. Less intense sessions burn fewer calories, but also place less stress and strain on your muscles, joints and other connective tissues, and still give a good endorphin rush to make you feel physically and mentally great.

THE JOY OF JOURNALING
There's huge swathes of science that suggest keeping a daily journal is as good for your mental health as following an exercise plan is for your physical health. And the best bit about journaling is that it's so easy to do: simply start by keeping a notebook and pen by your bedside table. Each night before you turn off the light, write down one thing for which you are truly grateful and the one key task you want to achieve tomorrow - that's it!

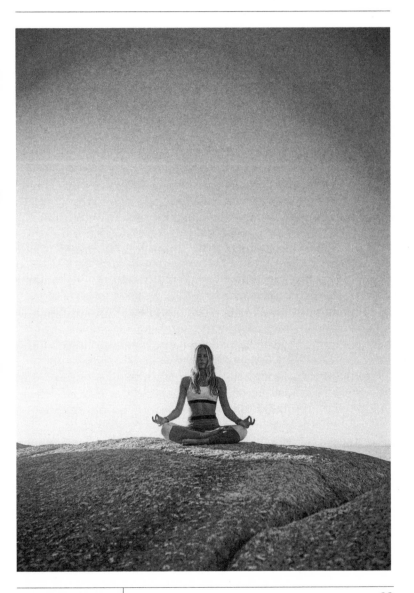

Sort your sleep

Sleep deeper for longer and build a better body

Sleep is one of the four critical pillars - alongside following a progressive exercise plan, having a smart and sustainable approach to eating, and minimising all sources of acute stress - when you're trying to build the foundations of your best-ever body. But for many people sleep is simply the thing they do at the end of the day when it's dark and they're tired, rather than the critical part of each and every day that has a profound impact on your overall health and fitness. After all, sleep is the only time your mind and muscles have to recharge, rejuvenate and recover. Here's how to guarantee better-quality sleep, every night, so you can get leaner, fitter and healthier.

CUT BACK ON COFFEE

If you drink too much caffeine - from coffee, tea, energy drinks or any other caffeinated beverages - too late in the day then the chances are you'll either struggle to fall asleep, or won't be able to stay asleep. That's because caffeine, the world's most consumed stimulant, has a half-life (or the time it takes for half the dose to be removed from your body) of around six hours, so hangs around hours after your last cup to keep your brain buzzing. Try to avoid caffeine after 12pm to give your body the time it needs to flush it out of your system.

PUT YOUR PHONE TO SLEEP

We're constantly surrounded by the glowing lights of smartphones, tablets, laptops and TVs. And while screen time is necessary for both work and relaxation, staring at a screen too close to bedtime makes it far harder for you to fall asleep. That's because all these electronic devices emit blue light, which your brain interprets as day light, and so slows down or shuts off the production of melatonin, a key hormone involved in making you feel sleepy and want your bed. Try staying away from all screens for at least 45 minutes before you want to go to bed to give your brain time to wind down and let melatonin work its magic.

Reading a book is your best bet, but if you have an e-reader
change the display settings to Night Time mode, which emits
non-disruptive red light instead.

SOLVE YOUR STRESS

There's nothing more certain to keep you tossing and turning all
night long that worrying about something. Whether it's a personal
or professional issue, stress and anxiety can be the worst enemy
of a good night's sleep. Whatever is keeping you awake, try this:
on a piece of paper write down - in a sentence or two - what you
worries are, then a single-sentence solution or some action points
you can make happen tomorrow to rectify the situation. It sounds
so simple but this 60-second act of writing it down and proposing
a solution can seemingly "shift" the problem out of your head for
long enough for you to fall asleep.

AVOID ALCOHOL

Alcohol is best avoided when you want to lose weight. It contains
lots of calories you don't need, and makes it much harder to eat
the right kinds of foods to fuel your better-body mission. What's
more, although you may think it induces feelings of tiredness (and
it may sometimes help you fall asleep faster), alcohol seriously
disturbs sleep quality by preventing your brain from entering the
deeper, restorative phases of sleep that are so important to your
well-being. Limit alcohol consumption to special occasions, and
alternate each boozy drink with a pint of water.

BLACKOUT YOUR BEDROOM

One of the best ways to fall asleep - and stay asleep - is to keep
your bedroom cool and dark. Blackout curtains are a must if
you live in a big town or city, while having a summer and winter
duvet (and fan if required in the hotter months) can make the
world of difference in keeping you and your room at the optimal
temperature for uninterrupted sleep.

Build healthier habits

Forge good habits to make life easier and happier

All of our daily behaviours take the form of a habit. Some of these regular routines are very good for you - brushing your teeth is important for good oral hygiene - but other habits are less beneficial: hitting the snooze button every morning will mean you always start your day late, stressed and constantly playing catch-up. Forging healthy habits is so important for a fit and balanced life because they reduce the amount of time and energy you have to spend each day fixing problems created by bad habits. Here are some of the best habits you can put into practice today to start feeling healthier and happier.

MAKE TIME TO MOVE

The physical and mental benefits of exercise are so profound that if we could replicate the effects in a pill it would prescribed to every person on the planet. There's the obvious physical effects - increased muscle mass, reduced body-fat levels, better cardiovascular fitness and heart and lung function, amongst much more - but the mental health benefits shouldn't be ignored. A good workout gives a sense of satisfaction hard to replicate in the rest of your daily life. So book your planned sessions into your diary just like you would any other important meeting - and then stick to the schedule.

DRINK MORE WATER

It sounds too easy to be effective, but increasing your intake of water - aim for two litres of water on non-training days, and three or more on training days - has been show to improve physical and mental well-being and performance. Staying adequately hydrated makes burning fat easier, improves focus, and can stave off sweet-tooth cravings. Always carry a bottle of water with you and sip from it constantly.

EAT MORE VEGETABLES

If you're looking for the single-most important dietary change you can make to improve how good you look, feel and perform it's this: start eating more vegetables. Veggies are packed with many of the essential micronutrients, such as vitamins, minerals, fibre and other compounds such as phytochemicals, that have numerous health-boosting qualities. Aim for two fist-sized servings of vegetables with every meal, and eat a wide range of different coloured veg, because each kind has a different nutrient profile.

GET YOUR STUFF TOGETHER

If you're always running late or constantly surprised by "forgotten" work deadlines or "unexpected" household bills then do yourself a huge favour by getting more organised. Doing so will reduce your everyday stress levels to make becoming healthier and happier much easier. It's as simple as putting out tomorrow's work clothes before you go to bed, planning your week's meals in advance, or keeping a folder with bills and other documents in a secure but accessible place.

BE MORE MINDFUL

Mindfulness can be a scary word for some people, but it simply means taking your time over some essential daily tasks to fully appreciate all the good things in your life. A great place to start is by being more mindful at mealtimes: instead of eating your dinner on the couch or in front of the TV, sit at the table. Then take a moment before each mouthful to anticipate then appreciate the smell, taste, texture and other qualities of each bite. This will help you slow down the speed at which you eat, and enable you to re-learn your body's hunger and fullness signals so you never over-eat and end up feeling stuffed, bloated and uncomfortable. This is one of the smartest strategies to start eating for a leaner body.

WORK ON YOUR RELATIONSHIPS

Despite a constant bombardment of notifications from multiple social media platforms, many people now feel more isolated and disconnected than ever. Make the time the stay connected - or to re-connect - with friends, family, former collegues and other acquaintances whose company you enjoy. Technology can be great, but real-world socialising can't be beaten.

FOCUS ON THE POSITIVES

It's so easy in this day and age to fall in to the very unhelpful habit of only ever focusing on what's not going to plan in our lives, rather than thinking about all the amazing things we have to be grateful for. Writing down one thing that you are happy about each day is a genuinely powerful tool for increasing feelings of positivity and can give you the motivation needed to keep making positive habit changes.